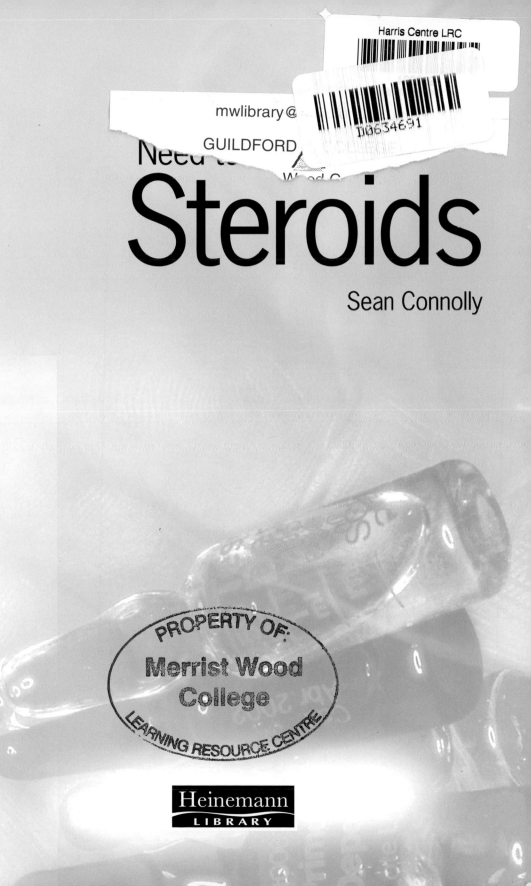

Need to

Steroids

Sean Connolly

Heinemann
LIBRARY

www.heinemann.co.uk

visit our website to find out more information about **Heinemann Library** books.

To order:

☎ Phone 44 (0) 1865 888066

📠 Send a fax to 44 (0) 1865 314091

💻 Visit the Heinemann Bookshop at www.heinemann.co.uk to browse our catalogue and order online.

First published in Great Britain by Heinemann Library, Halley Court, Jordan Hill, Oxford OX2 8EJ, a division of Reed Educational and Professional Publishing Ltd.

Heinemann is a registered trademark of Reed Educational & Professional Publishing Limited.

Oxford Melbourne Auckland Johannesburg Blantyre Gaborone Ibadan Portsmouth NH (USA) Chicago

Designed by M2 Graphic Design
Printed in Hong Kong / China
Originated by Ambassador Litho Ltd.

ISBN 0431 097828 (hardback)
04 03 02 01
10 9 8 7 6 5 4 3 2

ISBN 0431 097925 (paperback)
05 04 03 02 01
10 9 8 7 6 5 4 3 2 1

British Library Cataloguing in Publication Data
Sean Connolly
Steroids – (Need to know)
1. Steroids – Juvenile literature 2. Steroids – Physiological effect – Juvenile literature
I. Title 362.2'99

Acknowledgements
The Publishers would like to thank the following for permission to reproduce photographs: Allsport: pg.4, pg.5, pg.12, pg.21, pg.23, pg.29, pg.51; Body Builder: pg.7; Bubbles: pg.31, pg.48; Colorsport: pg.32, pg.42; Corbis: pg.40; David Hoffman: pg.6; Empics: pg.9; Hulton Getty: pg.16; Impact: Bruce Stevens pg.11, Rupert Conant pg.15, Caroline Penn pg.24; John Walmsley: pg.37; Rex Features: pg.19, pg.25; Science Photo Library: pg.13, pg.26, pg.33, pg.35, pg.39, pg.47; Telegraph Colour Library: pg.30; Zefa-Stockmarket: pg. 45.

Cover photograph reproduced with permission of David Hoffman.

Every effort has been made to contact copyright holders of any material reproduced in this book.
Any omissions will be rectified in subsequent printings if notice is given to the publisher.

Any words appearing in the text in bold, **like this**, are explained in the Glossary.

Contents

Introduction

The world of sport was blown apart in spectacular style in the summer of 1988 at the premier international sporting competition, the Olympic Games. The final of the men's 100 metre race, unofficially known as the sprint to decide the fastest man on Earth, was won by the Canadian Ben Johnson. He not only beat his top-flight rivals but smashed the world record in the process. Not long afterwards, however, this dramatic triumph turned to ashes when Johnson tested positive for **anabolic steroids**.

It emerged that his explosive speed had been achieved through long-term use of the drugs. He was stripped of his title and the medal, and was banned from the sport.

Murky legacy

The high-profile case of Ben Johnson had brought to light a problem that many in the sporting world had long recognized – the use of anabolic steroids as an aid to fitness and achievement. Johnson was not the first, or the last, to be banned because of their use but before him it was thought that the problem was confined only to people interested in bulking up their muscles. There were rumours that steroids use was widespread among weight-lifters and wrestlers, but the public remained largely in the dark about steroids.

As in so many such cases, however, the Johnson episode increased public awareness about a problem that had become widespread, even at the highest levels of competitive sport. Since then, new methods of detection have been developed but at the same time new techniques to evade detection have also sprung up.

More than cheating

Using anabolic steroids in competition amounts to cheating – no more, no less. More seriously, however, these drugs pose a serious health risk for those who use them, even in the short term. Young people are particularly endangered because steroids can limit the body's growth.

At the same time they build up a range of longer-term problems to be faced in adulthood. Because they are so often linked with gruelling training sessions, steroids are sometimes seen simply as a boost for performance, but the truth is that they encourage a variety of side-effects that can lead to serious illness or even death.

What are steroids?

Steroids are synthetic substances related to **testosterone**, the most powerful male **hormone**. Testosterone governs the development of the male sexual organs as a boy reaches maturity. As part of this process it sets off the 'masculinizing' effects of male **puberty**, such as the deepening of the voice and the increased growth of body hair. At the same time, testosterone begins building up the body, strengthening and encouraging the growth of muscle tissue.

Chemical echoes

Synthetically derived steroids also carry out these two functions. Nearly every known steroid leads to **androgenic** results, which correspond to the masculine side-effects of testosterone production. At the same time – and far more important to the people who take steroids – the **anabolic** effects echo the body-building role of the naturally-produced male hormones.

Pharmaceutical companies are constantly trying to produce steroids that are solely anabolic in their effect, without the androgenic aspects. There are many perceived advantages in taking such **anabolic steroids**, particularly in the world of sports and body-building.

Anabolic steroids often come in bottles, and the liquid can either be drunk or injected.

American body-builder Mike Mentzer opposes the use of anabolic steroids and has urged other body-builders to admit their use of steroids.

Users of anabolic steroids claim to become more aggressive and more willing to train harder. These results accompany the measurable changes in the user's body shape, with muscles becoming larger and more pronounced.

How steroids work

Although most people involved in sports and medicine agree that steroids do produce changes, it is difficult to analyze quite why these changes take place. Some analysts believe that once in the bloodstream, the drug seeks out cells with which it has a close relationship. These cells include many in the brain, in hair follicles and in particular in the muscles supporting the skeleton. After a series of chemical exchanges, the steroids enable the 'host' cells to produce more protein. In skeletal muscles, the results of increased protein production are evident in their enhanced size and bulk. In addition to these effects, steroids are also thought to increase the flow of blood throughout the body, enabling more oxygen to supply the muscles. They also seem to act against the effects of **cortisol**, which the body produces naturally to break down muscle mass and to control amounts of protein. Many of these normally 'controlled' proteins carry fat; reducing the controls puts pressure on the heart.

Are steroids addictive?

Using drugs for non-medical purposes leads to the important issue of addiction. Use of steroids involves none of the obvious images associated with addiction, such as needle-scars or chain-smoking. It is important, therefore, to establish just what addiction is and to identify different aspects of it.

Several medical texts define addiction as 'the repetitive, compulsive use of a substance that occurs despite negative consequences to the user'. This definition can be made more specific, to distinguish between two types of **dependency** – psychological and physical. Heroin and alcohol are examples of drugs that create both types of dependency in an addict: a physically dependent heroin addict begins to need more and more of the drug to feel 'normal'. An alcoholic can seem unable to contemplate life without excessive drinking – an example of psychological dependency. Certain chemicals in the brain, sometimes called the 'pleasure circuits', are activated by drugs that produce psychological dependency. Linked to the idea of physical dependency is the concept of **withdrawal** – symptoms of ill health that occur when an addict stops using a drug.

❝We see people not being able to see their lives falling apart, people trying to get off the drug and not being able to.❞

(Kenneth Yashkin and Herbert Kleber, Yale University)

Olympic weightlifter Adrian Popa of Hungary has shown that sporting success at the highest level can be achieved without **anabolic steroids.**

Are steroids addictive?

Weighing the evidence

Anabolic steroids do not fit easily into the normal definitions of addiction, for several reasons. The first is that they do not produce a pleasurable change in mood in the way, for example, alcohol or heroin do when a user takes them. It is true that aggressive behaviour is a common side-effect and might even be sought after by some users, but the prime reason for taking steroids is certainly not for their 'buzz'. This means that in the strictest definition they are not psychologically addictive. Likewise it is not common for a steroid user to wake up with a physical craving for the drug.

None of these factors, however, can alter the fact that taking steroids regularly will produce many of the effects of addiction. Although there is no mood-lifting rush when someone takes steroids, their outlook does change and they may display some of the characteristics usually linked to addiction. While there might be little physical craving for steroids, a person does undergo a number of unpleasant physical changes when the steroids are stopped.

Altered outlook

Enjoying repeated sporting success, or simply seeing a developing muscle structure, can act as a powerful reason to continue taking steroids. Since most people understand the serious medical complications involved, it brings home the last phrase of the medical definition: 'despite negative consequences to the user'. This masking of the harmful truth, or **self-delusion**, is common among addicts of many drugs. It is also related to the user's changed self-perception: watching a body expand almost grotesquely has been described by some researchers as 'reverse anorexia'. Just like sufferers from the eating disorder anorexia nervosa, many steroid users lose track of what a normal body really looks like. Similarly, a steroid user also loses track of what their body is capable of achieving without the drug: a lot of the 'progress' and 'development' might have taken place anyway.

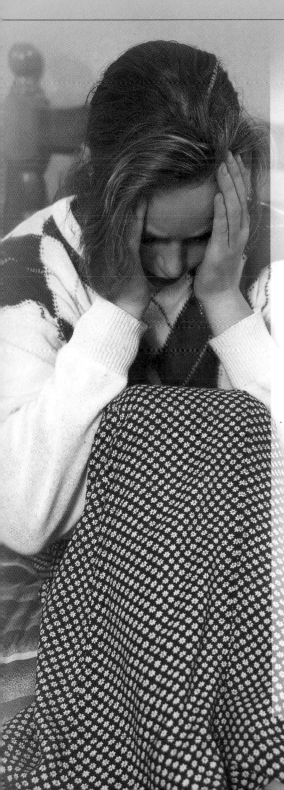

Case study

Although regular use of anabolic steroids falls short of the textbook definition of addiction, there have been some documented cases of steroid **dependence**. A case report published in 1989 provided evidence of a steroid user whose behaviour was addictive. After examining the subject for evidence of any of the nine categories designated by the American Psychiatric Association as being symptomatic of dependence, the scientists discovered six (exhibiting three for a month leads to a diagnosis of dependence). Among the symptoms shown were intolerance, an inability to reduce the dose and the use of steroids to avoid other symptoms such as irritability and depression.

Cold turkey

Withdrawal from an addictive drug usually produces a series of unpleasant physical side-effects, collectively known as 'cold turkey'. You may have seen films of heroin addicts or alcoholics suffering greatly when they have been denied access to the drug. Steroids seem to produce their own range of 'cold turkey' symptoms when users stop taking them. Among them are fatigue, depression, loss of appetite, sleeplessness and headaches. Some people have even considered suicide because of their violent mood swings as the effects of the steroids wears off.

Getting to know steroids

The **anabolic** – or 'body-building' – effects of taking steroids have lured many athletes over more than four decades, although using steroids is banned in most sporting competition and the trade in steroids is largely illegal. It is not hard to see why it might be tempting to try a 'quick fix' which could produce increased training power, personal bests and possibly even victory at the highest levels of sporting competition.

Taking steroids

Users take **anabolic steroids** either orally, in the form of pills and tablets, or by **intramuscular** injection.

A user will try to obtain properly produced steroids – which do have medical uses in combating **anaemia** and in strengthening chronically ill patients – although a multi-million pound **black market** also exists.

Typically, individuals use steroids over a fixed period of from six to twelve weeks. It is common for a user to combine – or **stack** – different types of steroids during this time. **Pyramiding** – steadily increasing the dose throughout the cycle – is also widespread. By the end of a cycle, some steroid users are taking doses that are up to 10 times those recommended for medical purposes.

The price to pay

Constant use of steroids produces a number of negative side-effects. Among men there is often a decrease in naturally produced **testosterone**, coupled with a shrinking of the testicles and a reduced **sperm count**. Women often undergo a number of 'masculinizing' changes, including increased growth of body hair, a deepening voice and even partial baldness. Steroids react strongly with oil-producing glands, so there is often a spread of acne in both sexes. Bad breath and swollen feet are other side-effects.

Most of these changes can be reversed if a person stops taking steroids, but there are also a number of irreversible changes. Long-term heavy use might cause permanent damage to the heart, liver and kidneys. Increased salt retention could trigger a heart attack. Young people must bear in mind that steroids are believed to send signals to the ends of bones to stop growing. A reduced adult height could be a high price to pay for temporarily bulked-out muscles.

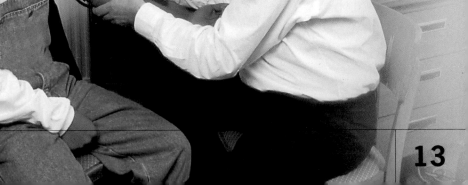

Getting to know steroids

Word of mouth

As is common among users of other illegal drugs, those people who take steroids learn about them – and how to obtain them – through the 'grapevine'. Typically, people who work out regularly in a public gymnasium or a health club become aware who is using steroids. Because of the 'underground' nature of steroid use, it is hard to tell exactly how many people use them.

Although it is difficult to gather hard evidence of the extent of steroid abuse, there have been some studies. One report, published in 1993, indicated that, of people who attended gyms regularly, up to 6 per cent of the men and 1.4 per cent of the women used steroids. What is clear, however – even without statistics – is that steroids seem more attractive to people involved in sports and pastimes that value strength and muscle bulk. Weight-lifting and body-building are the two most obvious examples.

Forbidden fruit

For some people the secrecy and illegality only add to the attraction of steroids. There are many well-documented accounts of sporting cheats who have been punished for using steroids to improve their performances. Although these stories have deterred many people from considering steroids, a minority of people are tempted to experiment with them, as long as they don't get caught. This temptation even extends beyond the immediate world of the athletes themselves. Coaches can also be lured by thoughts of rapid improvements among their team members.

"I wanted to be the best swimmer and the best black athlete ever."

(Grace, 17, former steroid user in the NIDA report on steroids)

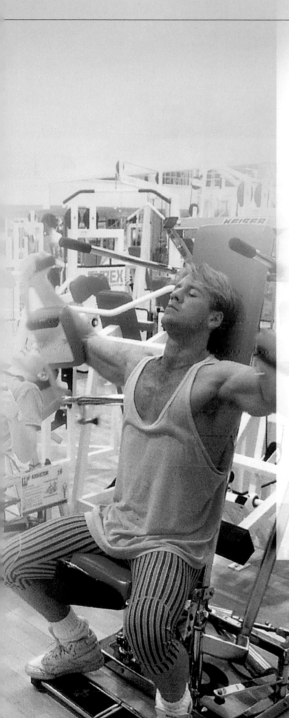

Innocent use of steroids

The illegal trade in **anabolic steroids** tries to tap into the flow of legally produced and distributed drugs that are used in the field of medicine. Steroids obtained on prescription from a registered chemist are used for a variety of medical conditions. Among them are the treatment of persistent **anaemia** where red blood cells cannot **regenerate**, the control of female **hormones** to limit the spread of breast cancer to secondary sites, the build up of protein in people recovering from surgery and treatment of some of the symptoms of the female **menopause**. The prescribed amounts of steroids in each of these cases is far lower than the amounts taken by those who use them for non-medical reasons. In addition, there are several types of steroids, known as corticosteroids, used for treating eczema and asthma. These are free of any **anabolic** side-effects.

The first steroids

Steroids entered the world of sport through activities such as wrestling, where increase of strength and body bulk are distinct advantages.

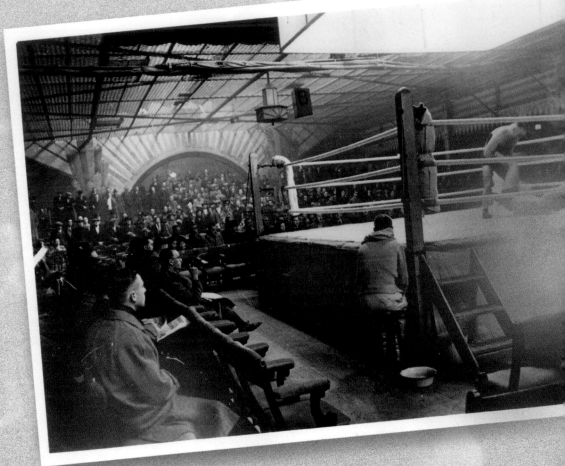

"The overwhelming majority of athletes I know would do anything and take anything short of killing themselves to improve athletic performance."

(Harold Connelly, 1956 Olympic hammer throw gold medallist)

Today's use, both legal and illegal, of **anabolic steroids** can be traced back to medical advances early in the twentieth century. At that time scientists had begun to understand the chemical structure and purpose of the many **hormones** produced by the human body. Various medical treatments were developed by isolating or chemically reproducing these hormones.

Testosterone is one of these medically useful hormones. It is present in small amounts in women but in far greater amounts in men, especially after **puberty**. At that stage in a young man's life testosterone is responsible for his sexual development as well as for the noticeable development of his muscles. More than 60 years ago medical researchers noticed that certain conditions, such as **anaemia** among men, could be treated with testosterone. These patients could not produce enough of the hormone on their own. Soon **pharmaceutical** companies were able to **synthesize** substances that were closely related to testosterone – anabolic steroids. The protein stimulation that was so helpful against anaemia also proved useful for helping patients who were weakened because of surgery or who had been through a long period when they were confined to bed. Steroids proved particularly useful in stimulating the growth of new tissue in burns patients. This stimulation highlighted the **anabolic** or body-building power of steroids.

Win at all costs

Word of these anabolic benefits spread through the medical world, and from there to the world of sport. A bulkier body, linked with a boost in strength, would be an advantage in many sports. By the 1950s there were reports of weight-lifters, wrestlers and field athletes improving their performances by taking steroids.

Several factors helped strengthen this 'win at all costs' attitude among athletes. The first was the dawn of **commercialism** in the world of sport, and with it the prospect of increased earning power tied in with victory. Another motive was political. The 1950s was one of the most fraught periods of the **Cold War**, when the United States and its western allies and the **Soviet Union** and its allies, known as the **Eastern Bloc**, were rivals for world leadership. This 'war' was fought on many fronts – even on the playing field. An Olympic gold medal began to mean more than an excellent individual performance; it was proof of a superior social system. Anabolic steroids provided a way to ensure that superiority.

The problem develops

From the first isolated cases of athletes using **anabolic steroids** for non-medical purposes in the 1950s, the world began to learn more about these substances and how people were using them to their own advantage. Lovers of true sporting competition were dismayed to hear of these 'artificially induced' improvements in a wide range of sports, with the possibility that further cheats had gone undetected. In addition, doctors had become aware of the practice of **pyramiding**, and with it the increased likelihood of dangerous side-effects.

Olympic response

In 1962 the International Olympic Committee (IOC) passed a resolution against **doping**, and it was worded to include the misuse of anabolic steroids. In the following year the Council of Europe adopted a clear definition of doping, paving the way for tests to be carried out on competitors. The first Olympic drugs tests were made in the 1968 Olympics, both in the Summer Games (in Mexico City) and in the Winter Games (in Grenoble).

These tests were not set up to detect steroids but there were positive results in several other drugs, suggesting that steroid tests might also have found positive results.

A new method of steroid detection, called gas **chromatography**, was developed in the early 1970s and the IOC was able to ban steroids in 1974. Earlier suspicions about steroid use were confirmed in the next Olympic Games (Montreal 1976), the first in which steroid tests were carried out. Eight weight-lifters tested positive. Here was proof that competitors were confidently taking steroids at the highest levels. However, the tests were carried out at specific dates and places, making it possible to mask the evidence of steroid use by coming off the drug in time. Fuller detection only came in the early 1980s when sports officials began carrying out random tests on competitors.

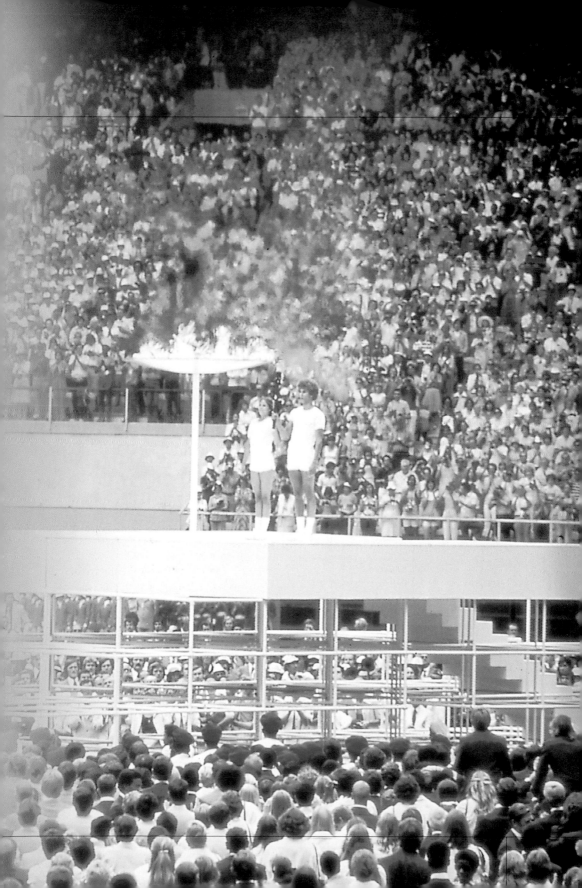

Tarnished gold

Positive **doping** tests in subsequent Olympic Games in the 1980s indicated that steroid use had moved on from its original 'body-bulk' sports, such as weight-lifting, shot put and hammer throw, into a wider range of pursuits. Selective use of steroids, coupled with specific training regimes, was entering the sporting arena in many other areas. Positive tests for volleyball (Los Angeles 1984) and ice hockey (Calgary 1988) were evidence of this new trend.

The biggest shock came in the 1988 Summer Olympic Games, held in Seoul, South Korea. The stage was set for the finals of one of the most high-profile events on the Olympic calendar – the men's 100 metre final, often described as a test to decide the fastest person on Earth. The Canadian sprinter Ben Johnson had broken the world record in 1987 and was set for a showdown against his arch-rival, the US sprinter (and 1984 gold medallist) Carl Lewis. Johnson flew past Lewis and the rest of the field, winning the gold easily. His time of 9.79 seconds also broke his own world record.

The shocking truth emerged not long after the Olympic Games had finished. An analysis of Johnson's urine indicated that he had been engaged in long-term **anabolic steroid** use. Johnson was stripped of his gold medal and banned from international competition for two years.

Lewis was awarded the title and the medal. He has remained a strong opponent of drug use. Johnson began competing again in 1991 but never recovered his previous world-class form. In 1993 Johnson was found to have been using steroids again and he was banned permanently from athletic competition.

Rica Reinisch of the former East Germany had been given anabolic steroids by her coaches from the age of 12. She went on to win three Olympic gold medals in swimming but now suffers from medical complaints related to drug use. She has now brought court action against those coaches.

Cold War competition

By the 1950s the United States and the **Soviet Union** were capable of destroying each other many times over with their **arsenals** of nuclear weapons. They needed to find other means of getting the upper hand. Psychological victories were vital to their cause, which is why both countries pumped billions of pounds into the 'Space Race' in the 1960s. They also used sporting achievement as a weapon in this war. Since the end of the **Cold War** in the early 1990s, there have been many reports of former widespread drug use in the **Eastern Bloc**, the group of European countries that were linked to the Soviet Union. East Germany, for example, produced far more Olympic medal-winners than many much larger countries. Many of these triumphs have since been tarnished by the news that they were achieved through the systematic – and possibly forced – use of anabolic steroids. Some East German swimmers were forced to take steroids in order to remain on the Olympic team; others did not even know that they were taking the drug.

Who takes steroids?

In the space of about fifty years use of steroids had moved on from its original, very specific, medical purpose and had begun to attract people who wanted to change their bodies in some way. Fuelled in part by commercial incentives to succeed in the sporting world, use of steroids became more widespread. Users tried to seek out new variations of steroids and ways to avoid detection. This 'cat and mouse game' has carried on throughout the quarter-century since the IOC banned steroids, but random testing seems to have dimmed the attraction of steroids for many athletes.

Athletic performance, however, is only part of the steroid story. For some people, the idea of bulking out a set of muscles can be an end in itself. Even the most inexperienced steroid user realizes that these drugs on their own do not improve muscles. The steroids work best on the muscles being exercised, as in a training session. Body-builders, for example, have traditionally worked certain sets of muscles repeatedly to achieve maximum size and mass. Imagine the temptation of being able to go even further without additional training.

Body-builders are not alone in being attracted to the idea of a new shape.

Doormen, security guards, prison officers and many others whose jobs may require a powerful appearance can feel the temptation to 'beef up' their image. An underground trade in steroids also exists within these circles.

Image problems

Most worrying, perhaps, is the idea of **anabolic steroids** becoming what many people describe as a 'lifestyle drug'. Impressionable young people, living in a world of designer sportswear and social rivalries, can feel tempted to change their image to appear tougher and more forceful. They also learn that steroids can increase a sense of aggression, leading to what are called **roid rages**. This is a play on the words 'road rage', which describe violent confrontations between drivers on the roads. Increased strength, coupled with artificially induced aggression and possibly alcohol, can create a frightening combination. Such steroid users are still very immature but they feel they are copying the 'up front' actions of prominent role models, whether they be action film stars, snarling boxers or footballers playing to the crowds after a goal. Many simply feel that these changed attitudes make them harder and more 'manly'.

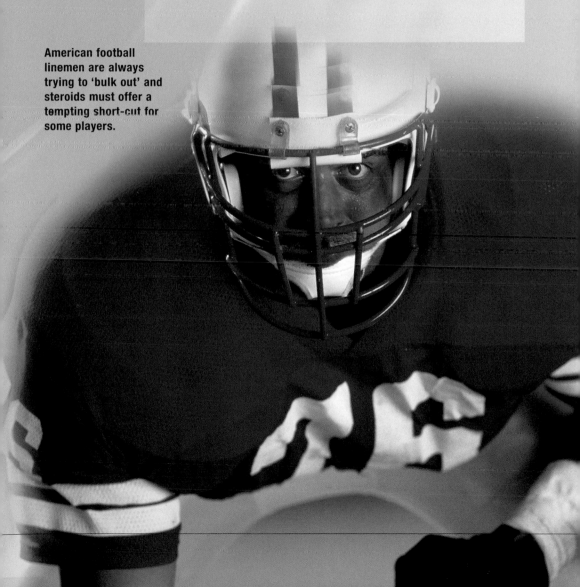

❝I preach to my team-mates all the time about living right. There is nothing that drugs do for you that is good for you. Whether it's steroids, cocaine or marijuana, it's all no good for you.❞

(Charlie Ward, star of the New York Knicks basketball team)

American football linemen are always trying to 'bulk out' and steroids must offer a tempting short-cut for some players.

Getting personal

Anabolic steroids were developed as a way of matching the function of the male **hormone testosterone**. This hormone is released constantly by the testes, and when steroids are prescribed medically doctors try to match this steady low level. The testosterone passing through the body acts to maintain muscle tone, rebuilding tissue where necessary. However, steroid abusers are not looking for a steady low level, they want dramatic increases in muscle bulk. That means taking more steroids than the body would normally process, in increasing amounts.

Building the pyramid

This increasing dosage, and the dramatic effects that it might supply, are known as **pyramiding**. The user takes larger and larger amounts of steroids over a period of weeks. Instead of taking a medically prescribed amount of perhaps 75–100 milligrams a week, the user could be taking a gram, which is ten or more times the prescribed amount.

Steroids can be taken either orally (in pill or tablet form) or by injection. Injectable preparations seem to cause less damage because – by avoiding the digestive system – they seem not to damage the liver as much as steroids taken orally. However, the body's system is able to clear away traces of orally taken steroids more quickly, making them harder to detect.

Leap into the unknown

Many aspects of using steroids remain mysterious – exactly how they work, how much is 'too much' and how specific the results of any single steroid will be. This medical grey area has given rise to word-of-mouth accounts that users pass on to each other. Pyramiding, based on the idea that more must be better, is one result. **Stacking**, or combining different steroid preparations with other drugs during a cycle, is another. This method is aimed at trying to increase the benefits of the steroids by minimizing the side-effects.

Typically, after the steroid training programme has been completed, the user stops using the drugs for several weeks so that the body can regain its natural balance. It is easy, however, to mistake certain changes, such as acne clearing up, for a permanent return to a balanced system. The seeds for longer-term side-effects have been planted, and will grow once steroids are taken again.

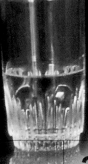

Increasing the risk

Long-term steroid users, and some medical researchers, have argued that there is definitely an extra edge to be had by building up doses in a **pyramiding** system. They argue that even if a certain level of steroids will attain maximum muscle-building effect, the extra steroids help by fighting the process of muscle breakdown. Such tissue breakdown is a normal bodily process, brought about by the hormone **cortisol**. Taking huge amounts of steroids might prevent the effects of cortisol, allowing continued muscle building with no natural trade-off. The obvious downside, of course, is that these huge amounts also magnify the known medical damage caused by steroid use.

Getting hold of steroids

Anabolic steroids come from two main sources. They are either legitimate medical preparations which have been diverted on to the **black market**, or they are manufactured and traded illegally. Legally produced supplies generally enter the black market through theft from **pharmaceutical** companies or through the criminal use of fake prescriptions. Steroids produced in secret laboratories carry no industry back-up: they are often very impure, adding to the dangers already present in steroid abuse.

Suppliers tend to gather around gyms and health clubs and other training venues. Even school playing fields are used.

Again, there are two main avenues for the flow of steroids. The first comprises people who are involved in the fields of medicine or sports, including coaches, fellow athletes, pharmacists or even doctors. Many users learn how to obtain and use steroids from an underground manual, or 'bible', that circulates in many western countries. In addition, a number of websites on the Internet provide information about supply and production of anabolic steroids. Unlike printed matter, this information is not subject to censorship. Most sites skirt the laws against illegal use of steroids by stating that they do not support all of the actions that appear on their site.

❝The site deals with today's body-building. We discuss the best training techniques, cutting edge supplements and the use of pharmaceuticals. This section of the site is an open forum and we do not take any responsibility as to the content of the message board since it is a public forum.❞

(Part of the disclaimer on a website)

Family and friends

Facing the facts

It is only when family members or friends begin to have suspicions that a steroid user has to confront their **self-delusion**. Parents might express concern that the training has become excessive, and that studies or relations in the home are suffering. Friends might also begin to feel left out of the user's life as working out and constant exercise become more dominant. There is less time for other pursuits and hobbies, such as music, films or simply socializing. This becomes a vicious circle, making the whole training regime seem all the more important. Even fellow members of a sports club or team can feel annoyed that their friend has gone so far down the road of obsessive exercise. Easy-going, well-rounded friends are often pushed out or replaced by other users who 'understand' the need to improve, improve, improve.

On top of all these comparatively subtle social effects there is the whole issue of the user's personality. Single-mindedness and determination are one thing – and most competitive athletes share these qualities – but regular steroid use produces intense bouts of aggression. These **roid rages** are unsettling for anyone who is fond of a user and knows the person's true character.

The steroid scene

Having been drawn into the use of steroids, many users begin to have some doubts. Their own changing behaviour may have robbed them of the chance to talk things through with family and friends. In this position, a user will often do what users of other drugs do – turn to other users for support and justification. The solitary world of constant training limits such contact, although a user may approach their supplier or other known users in the same club or gym. These people are unlikely to talk a user out of taking steroids. Instead, they will provide information about **stacking** or **pyramiding**, or simply about how to get hold of more supplies.

On average a user will pay about £20 for 100 tablets of the most common steroid preparations, although certain types, such as Deca-Durabolin and Sustanon, can cost £30 or more for ten vials. A typical steroid user spends about £40 a month on supplies.

❝I daydreamed about walking down the hall in short shorts and a tank top and a great tan.❞

(Mark, 15: NIDA Research Report)

The steroid scene

The teenage years are a complex and confusing time for most people, with difficult experiences and decisions to face nearly every day. The issue of drugs is one of the most troublesome of all these areas since it can be tied in with **peer pressure**, curiosity and rebellion. The issue of **anabolic steroids** complicates matters further, since, on the surface at least, it is linked with 'safe' pursuits such as sports and training. Self-image also plays a part in causing some people to experiment with steroids.

Relationships at risk

Many young people have a strong urge to prove themselves – to their immediate family, to their schoolmates and to their friends – yet these same relationships can become strained if a person starts using steroids regularly. Sometimes loved ones don't find out about a person's use of steroids until some serious damage has been done.

Unlike other drugs that young people sometimes use, such as alcohol, marijuana, ecstasy or amphetamines, anabolic steroids do not produce an immediate change in behaviour.

There is no obvious 'high' or 'buzz' which other people might recognize as a clue to drug use. In fact, many of the first effects of steroid use mimic the very achievements that normally signal a balanced lifestyle.

Eagerness to train, a developing and muscular body and sporting improvements are all seen as admirable elements in a young person's life. A steroid user can easily let unspoken praise from family members seem like an equally unspoken approval of the drug use.

Modern information and communications technology can be used in the illegal trade in steroids, and to detect irregular patterns of prescription.

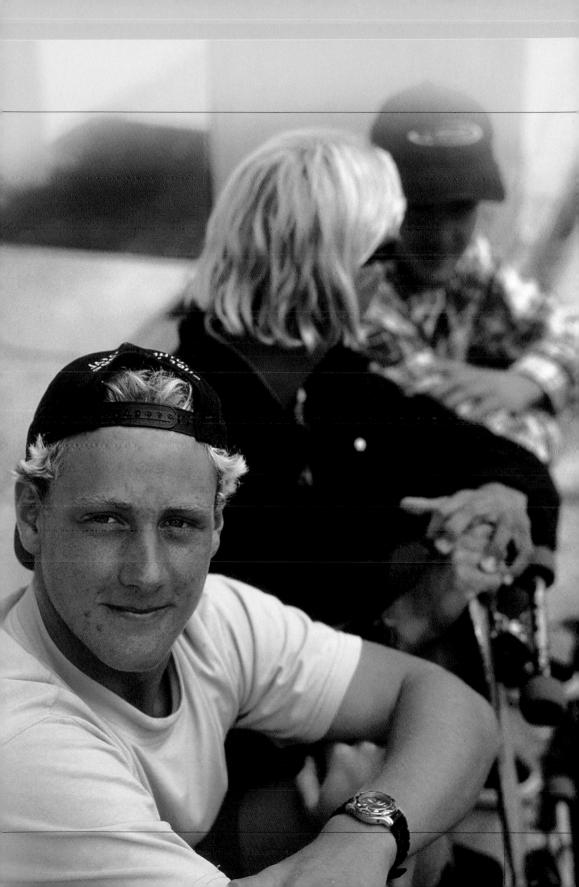

The steroid industry

The steroid scene

Anabolic steroids were originally developed – and continue to be used – for medicinal purposes. Controlled use of these drugs, under the supervision of a doctor, can lead to marked improvements in the condition of patients suffering from **anaemia**, low **testosterone** levels, burnt tissue or weakness caused by confinement. For this reason, steroids continue to be produced and distributed legally.

These accepted medical purposes for producing steroids emphasize the **anabolic** nature of the drug, since it is the 'building-up' side of the **hormone** that helps a patient's recovery. However, most synthetic steroids are derived from testosterone, which also plays an important **androgenic** role in helping a male body mature. Increased facial hair and a deepening voice are natural for an adolescent male, but they are unwanted side-effects for the vast majority of patients who have steroids prescribed.

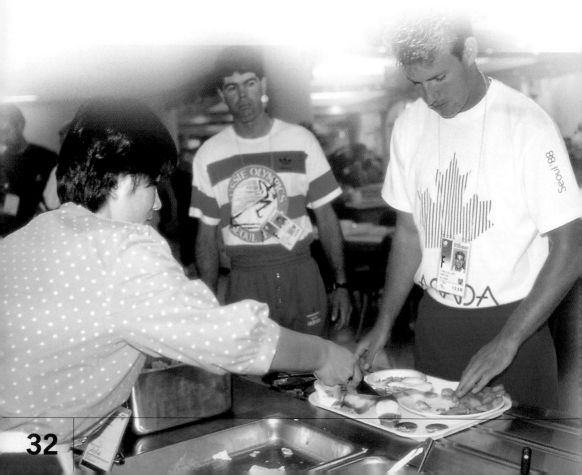

Continuing search

Knowing that the androgenic or **'virilizing'** side-effects of steroids are not wanted by women and children in particular, major **pharmaceutical** firms continue to search for a way of producing steroids that are almost exclusively anabolic in their actions.

So far, there has been no success in eliminating all of the androgenic properties, but all the research has led to a greater variety of steroid products on the market. Since the pharmaceutical industry, like other industries, is driven by competition and the search for profits, each new advance in steroid production is hailed as a breakthrough by the firm that develops it. All of this can lead to some confusion, even among doctors who prescribe steroids. More ominously, a new steroid formula can also be just what a steroid cheat is looking for since such an athlete might feel they have scored a point against existing dope-testing methods.

Corticosteroids

It's not uncommon for a doctor to prescribe steroids for a patient who is suffering from asthma, eczema or even arthritis. Many patients react with alarm to the word 'steroid', but this group of steroids is different from anabolic steroids, both in chemical make-up and in its effects on the body. Such steroids are usually part of a group known as corticosteroids, which occur naturally or are **synthesized** to resemble those produced in the human body. Often taken in aerosol form, these steroids have none of the virilizing effects of those steroids based on testosterone.

Asthma inhalers often contain corticosteroids, which have none of the dangerous side-effects of anabolic steroids.

33

The black market

Continuing search

With strict controls on the prescription and use of steroids, coupled with the lure of the forbidden, it is not surprising that a large **black market** operates outside the legitimate steroid industry. What began some fifty years ago as the occasional bottle of tablets sneaked to a power athlete or body-builder has developed into a sophisticated worldwide operation, trying to keep one step ahead of the authorities. It is estimated that the illegal trade in steroids is worth US$400 million a year in the United States alone, and most developed countries could give similarly alarming figures.

Strict safeguards

The most reliable source of steroids, from the user's point of view, is through legitimate channels, or a supplier operating as closely as possible to these channels. In order for steroids to be distributed in this way, someone within the legitimate industry must be prepared to lie, steal or defraud a company. Knowing that their products have this unethical lure, and in the interests of maintaining profits, **pharmaceutical** companies keep detailed records of the flow of steroids at every stage of production, from testing and research right through to distribution to medical authorities. Any employee caught siphoning off a supply of steroids faces dismissal or even criminal charges.

Similar safeguards operate within the medical world. It would take an incredibly foolish doctor, nurse or laboratory technician to risk their professional standing by becoming involved in the black market for steroids. Veterinary surgeons, who can prescribe steroids for animals, are similarly held back by ethical and professional concerns. Faced with the overwhelming evidence that a lucrative black market does exist, we are faced with the question: where do the illegal steroids come from?

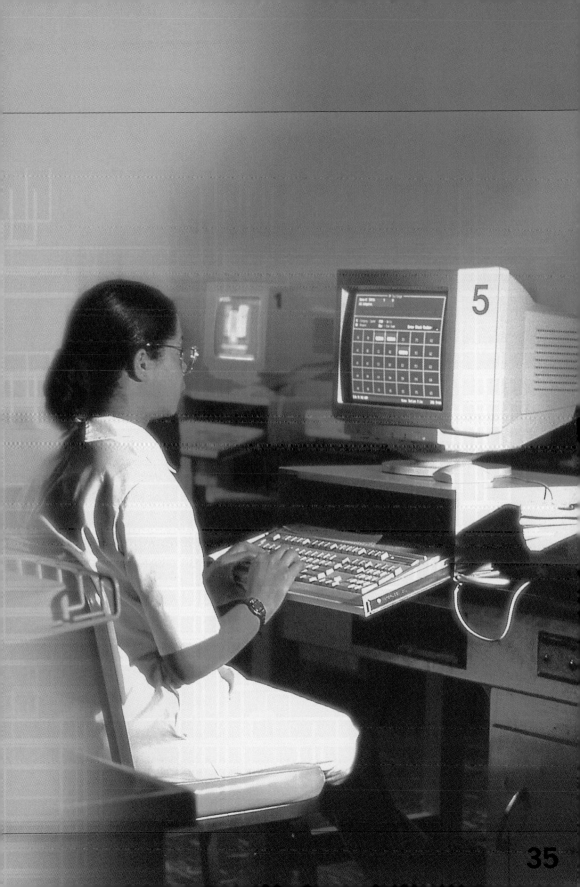

Secret labs

The simple answer is that most steroids sold outside accepted prescription channels are fake, and not made in legitimate **pharmaceutical** company laboratories. Instead, such counterfeit steroids are made in 'underground labs' and sold as the real thing. Apart from the illegal nature of these labs, a number of serious concerns arise from this process. The first is to do with the qualifications of the 'scientist' producing these drugs. Absolutely no safeguards exist to maintain any health or pharmaceutical standards. Likewise there are no industry 'watchdogs' to monitor hygiene, ingredients or dosages, all of which are scrupulously observed within the pharmaceutical industry.

These behind-the-scenes activities give rise to a bewildering array of products. The counterfeit drug industry predates the rise in steroid demand and the secret labs use all the known tricks used in producing and distributing other 'home-made' drugs such as LSD, ecstasy, cocaine. As a result the potential buyer faces a number of risks above and beyond those associated with genuine steroids.

The illegal steroid buyer must therefore be prepared for 'steroids' that:

- have little or no steroid content at all
- have more than the dose indicated on the bottle
- have less than the dose indicated on the bottle
- are different from the type of steroid indicated on the bottle.

Such uncertainty should be enough to deter anyone from tampering so dangerously with their own health. Unfortunately, people still do.

Maintaining the image

Those people who deal in illegal steroids – as well as those who pass on legitimately produced versions – rely on the gullibility of the people who intend to buy. A teenage boy with posters of sports heroes on his bedroom wall, an ardent body-building enthusiast, or an athlete looking for that extra 'edge' – all are fair game for a glamorous campaign of misleading or false information. None of this information, being illegal in nature, is passed on through normal advertising on television, radio or newspapers.

Instead, those interested in promoting widespread use of steroids spread 'success stories' by word of mouth, usually linked with reassuring advice on how to avoid developing any side-effects or being caught. Underground publications strengthen this message and are sometimes seen at gyms or health centres.

Even more commonly, people find information about steroids through a large number of websites on the Internet. These sites often start with a declaration that they 'in no way endorse the illegal distribution or use of **anabolic steroids'** and then go on to give specific advice on dose levels, **stacking** and **pyramiding.**

Some young people find it easy to be swayed by those who claim that steroids are safe and acceptable.

Medical fallout

Many of the unwanted side-effects of using steroids become clear soon after someone begins using them regularly. As mentioned earlier in this book, these effects can range from cosmetic changes such as acne and weight gain through to more serious consequences such as hair loss, water retention (which puts a strain on the heart) and reduced sex drive. More worrying, and often irreversible, changes also lie in store. Teenagers run the serious risk of stunting their growth, while there are increased risks of heart disease, liver failure and the danger of miscarriage during pregnancy.

Leap into the unknown

These same risks are magnified when the user has a supply of counterfeit steroids. With dosages hard to monitor accurately, coupled with the likelihood of **stacking** and **pyramiding**, most users are taking a trip into the unknown. Studies have also shown that subtle psychological changes occur with steroid use: the more a user sees changes in their own body, the more attractive such changes seem to be. This altering of perception can lead to longer spells of steroid use or larger doses during a steroid cycle. Worst of all, the user generally denies that these changes have occurred.

The needle and the damage done

On top of all these adverse medical consequences, some steroid users dance with death. Many users believe that steroids taken orally are more damaging to the liver and that injected steroids are therefore safer. However, a drug user who injects will often be tempted to share a needle with another user. Conditions are rarely sterile and users can expect to develop sores or abscesses – and blood poisoning – as a result. Sharing needles also introduces the risk of spreading blood-borne diseases such as **HIV** or **hepatitis** B or C, with potentially fatal consequences.

Safety delusions

Rumour and hearsay counts for a lot in the general use of steroids, and many people feel they can escape ill-effects by following snippets of advice heard through the grapevine. For example, women sometimes feel that injecting steroids in controlled, sterile conditions will lead to less overall harm. However, research suggests that the opposite is true for women – oral preparations cause less harm because they do not linger as long in the body. Even with this form of steroids there are problems that user 'friends' might not have told them. A woman's liver – the organ commonly damaged by steroids – is smaller than a man's, so the damaging effects of any type of steroid are magnified.

Steroid use is as likely to lead someone to the intensive care unit as it is to boost them onto the winner's podium.

Legal matters

The past few decades have seen a crackdown on the use of **anabolic steroids** in nearly every competitive sport played at any level. Increasingly sophisticated testing procedures, coupled with random testing of athletes involved in competitions, have helped make the ban on steroids stick. Competitors face punishments ranging from warnings to suspensions and even lifetime bans. The reasons for the ban on steroids, and for the strict measures to enforce the ban, are twofold. First, there are serious concerns about the medical effects of using steroids. Second, the simple fact is that using steroids is cheating, every bit as much as putting iron blocks in boxing gloves would be.

Former heavyweight boxer Bob Hazelton has lost both legs because of many years of steroid use.

The legal view

In addition to the disciplinary procedures for steroids in the sporting world, there are strict legal restrictions on the possession and supply of **anabolic steroids**. In the UK, two Parliamentary Acts define the British legal position. The first is the 1968 Medicines Act, which stipulates that steroids can only be sold by a pharmacist working from a registered pharmacy and then only on the presentation of a doctor's prescription.

The second law is the Misuse of Drugs Act 1971 (MDA), which puts anabolic steroids in the Class C category. This classification means that simple possession of steroids is not illegal (since they can be prescribed), but that the illegal supply of the drugs does carry strict penalties. In the UK, when someone is caught with illegal drugs, the police must take one of the following actions. They can either issue a Reprimand or a Warning to 10-17 year olds, or if the person is over 17 they can issue an Adult Caution. Or the police can decide to charge the person with an offence.

The sentence served by someone convicted of supplying steroids depends on their age. Up to the age of seventeen, people are tried in a young offenders' court, which can give a maximum sentence of one year in a young offenders' institution. People who are eighteen or older go through the **magistrates' courts** which can impose longer sentences, although until someone is twenty-one they still serve the time in a young offenders' institution.

In Australia the Australian Sports Drug Agency and the Australian Sports Drug Testing Laboratory in Sydney have IOC accreditation to carry out drug testing. A positive test result in fines and/or bans from participation for varying lengths of time.

The Misuse of Drugs Act

As the old saying goes, ignorance is no defence in a court of law. In the case of steroids and most controlled drugs, the law in question is the Misuse of Drugs Act 1971, which divides drugs into three classes and gives guidelines for penalties. Class A drugs, which include cocaine, crack, heroin and LSD, are considered most serious and the penalty for supply can be life imprisonment. Cannabis and speed (amphetamines) are considered Class B drugs, which carry up to fourteen-year prison sentences for supply. Supplying steroids and tranquillizers, although considered the least serious category (Class C), can still lead to a criminal record or a prison sentence and fine.

Life with steroids

Even knowing the extensive medical side-effects of taking steroids, as well as the legal risks involved, some people carry on taking these substances and others begin the same process. Why is this? The answer seems to be that although steroids produce largely physical results, it is psychological reasons that underlie a 'life with steroids'.

The roots of these psychological motives run deep within most people and include the desires to excel, to win prizes or simply to feel good about oneself. For most people, acting on these desires usually takes the form of following a good diet, regular exercise regimes, lively competition and good grooming. Other people either feel comfortable enough about themselves, or are too lazy to do anything besides get on with life.

Czech tennis star Peter Korda has not taken steroids, although in 1998 he tested positive for Nandrolone, a by-product of anabolic steroids. Korda was cleared by the International Tennis Federation after arguing that he was unaware that the Nandrolone was an ingredient in a training preparation he took.

A chosen lifestyle

Steroid users are different. Although many would deny it, they are using steroids as a crutch or boost in the same way that someone might try to solve problems with tranquillizers or amphetamines. Performers in the field of sports and body-building can be somewhat self-obsessed, and this type of drug use can become accepted and even turn into a lifestyle in itself.
A good example is Neal Brunning, a former international shot-putter who received a four-year British ban in 1992 after testing positive for steroids. Brunning was already a successful athlete before he considered taking steroids. But after a defeat in December 1991, at a competition where he felt other competitors were on steroids, he decided he needed an extra edge: 'I thought, "If everyone else can do it, why can't I? If they can do it and get away with it, then let's have a go."'

From December 1991 until February 1992, when he tested positive, Brunning was taking **testosterone**. Like many other steroid users, he had no real thoughts about the physical consequences as he saw his performances improve: 'I just wanted to get to the top. I don't think anyone cares if they think there's a chance of doing that.'

Tunnel vision

Brunning's experience echoes that of many other steroid users. He saw the drug as a performance enhancer. He also needed it to give him the stamina to train for long hours, even after his thirteen-hour working days as a chef. Like others, he used the drug with no real guidance and with no eye on the future. 'I didn't get any advice about what I was doing. I just took the tablets. I thought, "If I get caught, I get caught."' Results were all that mattered, but the only real result was the positive test in 1992 which put paid to his shot-putting career.

Life with steroids

Life as a steroid user

Neal Brunning is candid about his steroid use in the past. He now has nothing to do with drugs. He has even made a dramatic switch, and returned to compete in a new sport, judo. While he can thank his stars that his steroid-taking lapse ended so quickly, only two months after it began, others might not be so lucky.

Mark, a young body-builder from Oxford, was candid about his involvement with steroids when he was interviewed by the *Today* newspaper in 1995. He was preparing to take 500 milligrams of testosterone, a weekly amount that would build up by **pyramiding** to 2000 milligrams a week in the course of his two-month steroid cycle. Coupled with his normal strenuous work-outs, the steroids would build his body from a normally powerful fourteen-stone frame to seventeen stone.

Mark felt secure that he could carry on using steroids, despite the criticisms of his doctor and his brother, an anti-drugs campaigner. Like Neal Brunning, he associated with people who tolerated, or even used, steroids. Referring to others at his local gym, he said, 'I reckon about 50 per cent of the lads are on steroids.'

In such a world, with a steady supply of steroids and without the testing and punishment that athletes like Neal Brunning face, individual users such as Mark run a far greater risk of doing serious damage to themselves.

❝I was going to get married but that split up. I had been thinking 100 per cent about athletics. I didn't care about anyone else – I blanked them out – and that was wrong.❞

(Neal Brunning, former shot-putter who served a four-year ban for using steroids)

"It's too easy to place the blame on others and point the finger at the Eastern Bloc. But the West also played a major part in the deceit and there are many athletes, now safely retired, who are basking in the glory they achieved through cheating, safe in the knowledge that they now will never be caught."

(Dave Moorcroft, former world 5000-metre record-holder)

Treatment and counselling

Very often the people who most need help with steroids are those who refuse to believe that there is a problem in the first place. Rippling muscles, increased self-esteem, sporting success and peer approval are undoubtedly reasons for people to believe that they are on to a winner with steroids. So it is also the failure to recognize the problem – like the alcoholic's claim that 'just one drink won't hurt' – that works against any treatment.

Hiding the truth

Other obstacles relate to the steroids themselves. Because the steroids that are abused are spin-offs from legitimate, evolving **pharmaceutical** research there are new variants appearing constantly on the **black market**. Abusers are very rarely truthful about the amounts that they take – including amounts of well-known steroids such as pure **testosterone** – so it can be hard for the medical profession to devise clear-cut strategies about dealing with the problem.

Doctors, chemists and other health workers are sometimes the only people who can work out that someone is abusing steroids.

Tied by rules of patient confidentiality, they know that it is a tricky job to set people on a healthier course. Presenting hard medical evidence – for example, about stunted growth in adolescents or reduced **sperm counts** in men – sometimes works. However, other approaches can backfire. For example, telling a young user about violations committed by well-known stars can simply promote the perceived performance-enhancing benefits of steroids.

The 'addiction' view

These strategies concentrate on the psychological side of steroid use. Other approaches deal more directly with the physical nature of steroid abuse, treating it as substance abuse. These approaches take into account some psychological aspects of steroid abuse, including mood swings, **roid rages** and distorted views about the user's body, but see them as part of a physical **dependence** or addiction.

Other features of steroid use add weight to this 'addiction' approach. When users are deprived of steroids during an intensive training programme, they often suffer from cravings and decreased self-esteem, which are classic symptoms of 'cold turkey'.

More evidence – again dependent on emerging medical research – suggests that **anabolic steroids** produce biological complications in the body similar to those associated with cocaine or alcohol abuse.

Some health clinics use the addiction approach as the basis for a course of treatment for steroid users.
Using techniques that have proved successful in other substance-abuse treatment programmes, they set about forcing the user to admit the exact scale of their use. Building on that, the clinics provide non-steroid alternatives to help maintain self-esteem or at least a sense of mental balance. These include the drugs clonidine and naloxone, and the user spends up to a week in the clinic under close observation. Often the physical craving and mental disturbance caused by stopping steroid use have stopped by this time, and both user and health officials can look to the longer term.

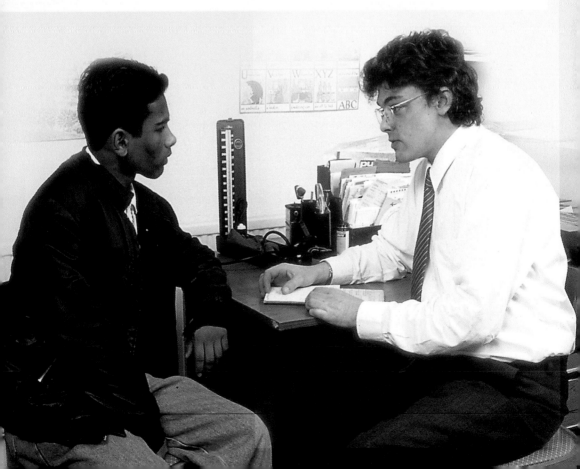

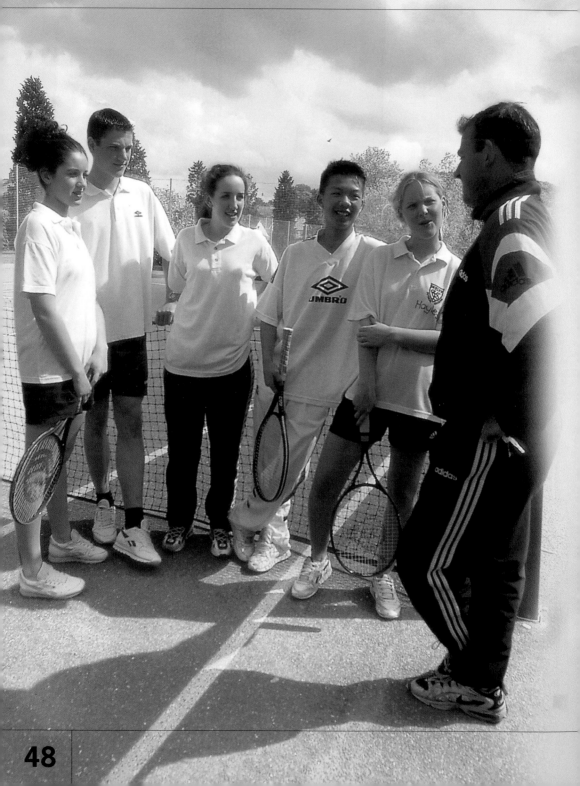

Follow-up

For whatever reason someone finally confronts a problem with steroid use – perhaps following a doctor's advice, accepting it as an addiction to be dealt with in a clinic or simply taking a personal course of action – a long-term follow-up is essential. The clearest indication that an end is in sight is when a former user believes their goals can still be achieved without the need for drugs.

A therapist's view

Ellen is a physical therapist with a health clinic in Wiltshire, England. She works with a team that deals with a wide range of physical ailments and complaints, ranging from chronic conditions such as arthritis, back problems and asthma, to acute problems such as fractured bones and muscular strains. Many of the acute problems are sports-related, and the patients that see her are sometimes steroid users.

'The biggest problem we face is one of denial, rather like the sort you might expect from an alcoholic who admits to having only the odd glass of wine,' she says. 'We can see – particularly in those patients who come here regularly – some of the classic signs of steroid abuse. We'll have someone in for, say, a muscle strain and during a massage they open up about their devotion to training.

A few weeks later we might see them again, boasting about some personal best or simply looking a lot more bulked out. That's when you think, "Hang on – there's more to this than just bench presses."'

Like others in the health profession, though, Ellen feels that the tactful approach is the best way to get to the heart of the problem. 'I know it doesn't sound like much, but sometimes a word or two about someone else's steroid side-effects can set them thinking. We're not like the Betty Ford Clinic (a US clinic for dealing with alcohol and drug problems), so we can't intervene directly with long-term, in-house treatment. But what we can do – and this is important – is to get the person to recognize that they've taken a wrong turning. You'd be surprised how many people own up and ask about where to turn for alternatives.'

People to talk to

Most people who get involved with steroids do so within some sort of framework or organization. It might be a team or sports club, a gym or a health club. Taking steroids might seem like a personal choice, but there is ample scope to talk things through with people who know a great deal about them. For anyone needing to know more about steroids, the best advice is talk – and listen. One of the most serious problems about drugs, including steroids, is secrecy.

Ground-level help

It would be stupid to suggest that there are no people out there who will advocate using steroids. Hear them out, but remember to ask yourself why they are taking that view. Do they have your best interests at heart, or are they trying to excuse their own use? Maybe they simply want to make money by supplying these drugs illegally.

Talk things through with a PE instructor or, if you are part of a team, ask your coach. People who are closely involved with the sporting world have a surprising amount of experience in dealing with steroid use.

If you are curious about the physical consequences of using steroids, ask a doctor or health professional. A professional in the world of sport or medicine can outline a sound fitness programme that has nothing to do with drugs.

High-profile examples

While there are plenty of people in any community who can offer sound advice about steroids and the problems associated with them, it is also worth noting that most successful sports stars have no need for drugs. Many, such as athletes Colin Jackson and Sally Gunnell and basketball star Michael Jordan, have made many public statements about the risks of drug use.

Many who are tempted to use steroids are driven by a force within themselves rather than a desire to copy others. These people should try to talk to others who have had first-hand experiences with steroids, and who will understand the urge to build up and become more powerful. If they are frank with themselves, they will be the best people to spell out the convincing reasons for staying clear of these powerful drugs.

Basketball legend Michael Jordan shattered records and led his team to several championships – while remaining an outspoken critic of all drug use in sport.

Information and advice

There are many organizations in the field of sports and drug awareness that can provide detailed information or confidential advice about the use of anabolic steroids and other drugs. If you want specific information relating to a sport not listed below, contact the Sports Councils in England, Scotland and Wales for contacts with the governing bodies of the sport in that particular region.

Sporting contacts

Sports Council Doping Control Unit
Walkden House, 3–10 Melton Street,
London, NW1 2EB
Tel: 020 7383 5667
The unit has a good range of leaflets and other publications on drugs in sport, including their own Drugs Information Pack.

The Football Association Medical Education Centre
Lileshall Hall National Sports Centre
Near Newport, Shropshire TF10 9AT
Tel: 01952 605 928
The Medical Education Centre has detailed information about the illegal use of drugs in football as well as useful contacts for information on other sports.

The Sports Council
16 Upper Woburn Place, London WC1H 0QP
Tel: 020 7388 1277
www.english.sports.gov.uk
The Sports Council has a wide range of information on all sports-related issues, including drugs. Similar listings are available for Scotland, Wales and Northern Ireland (addresses of their headquarters are provided below).

The Scottish Sports Council
Caledonia House, South Gyle
Edinburgh EH12 9D
Tel: 0131 317 7200

The Sports Council for Wales
Sophia Gardens, Cardiff CF1 9SW
Tel: 02920 300 500

Sports Council for Northern Ireland
House of Sport, Upper Malone Road
Belfast BT9 5LA
Tel: 01232 381 222, www.sportni.org

UK Athletics
Tel: 0121 456 5098
www.ukathletics.org
The national-level headquarters for athletics in the UK provides information on all aspects of the sport as well as links to regional governing bodies.

Drug awareness contacts

ISDD (Institute for the Study of Drug Dependence) Waterbridge House, 32-36 Loman Street London SE1 OEE, Tel: 020 7928 1211 www.isdd.co.uk
The ISDD has the largest drugs reference library in Europe and provides leaflets and other publications. SCODA (the Standing Committee on Drug Abuse) is located at the same address (tel: 020 7928 9500) and is one of the best UK contacts for information on drugs.

National Drugs Helpline Tel: 0800 776 600
The Helpline provides a free telephone contact for all aspects of drug use and has a database covering all of the British Isles for further information about specific drugs or regional information.

Contacts in Australia

ADCA, PO Box 269, Woden, ACT 2606 www.adca.org.au
The Alcohol and other Drug Council of Australia (ADCA), based in the Capital Territory, gives an overview of drug awareness organizations in Australia. Most of their work is carried out over the Internet but the postal address provides a useful link for those who are not 'on-line'.

Australian Drug Foundation, 409 King Street, West Melbourne, VIC 3003, Tel: 03 9278 8100 www.adf.org.au
The Australian Drug Foundation (ADF) has a wide range of information on all aspects of drugs, their effects and the legal position in Australia. It also provides handy links to state- and local-based drug organizations.

Centre for Education and Information on Drugs and Alcohol, Private Mail Bag 6 Rozelle, NSW 2039, Tel: 02 9818 0401 www.ceida.net.au
The Centre for Education and Information on Drugs and Alcohol is the ideal contact for information on drug programmes throughout Australia. It also has one of the most extensive libraries on drug-related subjects in the world.

Further reading

Buzzed, by Cynthia Kuhn, Scott Swartzwelder and Wilkie Wilson; New York and London: W.W. Norton and Company, 1998

Drugs, by Anita Naik, part of Wise Guides Series; London: Hodder Children's Books, 1997

Drugs and Violence in Sport, edited by Craig Donnellan; Cambridge: Independence, 1995

Drugs Wise, by Melanie McFadyean; Cambridge: Icon books, 1997

Taking Drugs Seriously, A Parent's Guide to Young People's Drug Use by Julian Cohen and James Kay; London: Thorsons, 1994

The Score: Facts about Drugs, HEA leaflet; London: Health Education Authority, 1998

Glossary

anabolic
causing (the body) to retain nitrogen, a basic element of protein, and leading to muscular bulking and extra strength

anabolic steroids
substances, either naturally occurring as male hormones or synthesized, that add muscle bulk and increase strength

anaemia
a medical condition caused by a reduced number of red blood cells and leading to paleness, weakness and breathlessness

androgenic
relating to the 'masculinizing' effects of male hormones, including a deepening voice and increased body hair

arsenal
a supply of weapons

black market
the illegal trade in something, such as drugs

chromatography
separating substances by absorbing them into paper or gas

Cold War
the period lasting roughly 45 years after the Second World War when the United States and its capitalist Western allies competed for world influence with the Soviet Union and its communist allies

commercialism
viewing something mainly as a way of making money

cortisol
a naturally occurring hormone that breaks down excess muscle tissue

dependence/ dependency
the physical or phychological craving for something

doping
using drugs illegally, especially as a way of cheating in sport

Eastern Bloc
the Eastern European countries that sided with the Soviet Union during the Cold War

hepatitis
illness associated with the liver, which can be fatal

HIV
Human Immunodeficiency Virus, which is linked with the disease AIDS

hormone
a chemical substance that is produced by the body and affects the function of specific organs when transported there by bodily fluids

intramuscular
taken (as a drug) under the skin and directly into a muscle, as in an injection

magistrates' court
a court that deals with legal cases involving relatively minor crimes

menopause
the period in a woman's life when she undergoes a number of physical changes corresponding with the end of her ability to have any more children